This book is by Diane Holliday who holds the copyright

This book is dedicated to my sister, Patricia Wynne
who introduced me to EFT

Contents

how To Use This Book	4
Abandonment	6
Abundance	9
Addictions	11
Allergies	13
Anger	15
Anxiety	17
Bereavement	19
Business And Career Issues	21
Cancer And Other Serious Illnesses	23
Children's Behavioral Issues	25
Chronic Fatigue Syndrome	27
Depression	29
Fears & Phobias	31
Fibromyalgia	33
Hypertension (High Blood Pressure)	35
Insomnia	37
Pain Management	39
Relationship Issues	41
Stress	43
Trauma (Ptsd) Post Traumatic Stress Disorder	45
Weight And Food Issues	47

This little book aims to fill a gap; to help you find the words and phrases when working with EFT (Emotional Freedom Techniques) by yourself.

I have been a practicing therapist and coach for many years and love EFT for its immediacy and ease of use, but I see a need for a resource which can become a pocket reference with just some words and phrases which will help you when stuck and trigger your own thoughts and words.

If you have been to see an EFT Practitioner or have been watching EFT DVDs, you no doubt have the tapping points embedded in your memory. But as many of my clients tell me, there is some difficulty in remembering the words. In my case I 'help' my clients to find the right words; at the start we use the words and phrases that come from the initial chat when we are focusing on the issue in hand and sometimes I may add a word or phrase and ask, "Is that true?" If it is then we use it.

The difficulty seems to be when we re-frame the issue and turn it on its head. So, this little book is designed to help you when you are working on your own and need reminding of some new words and phrases to help you find and eliminate your issues once and for all.

HOW TO USE THIS BOOK

In all cases I have assumed that you understand the principles of EFT (you can find all this on the FREE articles page of my web site) so have dispensed with the need to write each stage of the tapping points.

So, for instance, if you are suffering from Anxiety, you can look it up to find the appropriate words and phrases to access the issues and more words that you can use to re-frame and clear the issues you have found.

You only need to use the words that YOU find fit well with YOUR particular issues, so I would suggest that you underline the words and phrases that have the most meaning for you and then start the tapping routine.

You may also like to add your own phrases to the book in the space provided, so you can repeat the exercise at a later date. This is useful when new aspects arise and it's a good place to write your SUDS rating (0-10 intensity) and just watch it go down!

You may not find your issues listed so a little analysis may be required. Think about how you feel and break it down into smaller components. For instance, if you are fed up at work and feeling undervalued, you may need to work on anger, career related issues, stress and depression.

If you are constantly feeling ill then you may want to see your local medical doctor to ascertain what's going on, then when you have the details, work on that. Being always ill with one thing or another could have links to childhood, relationships or work issues that you have not yet addressed.

Don't forget to rate the emotional intensity on the scale of 0 to 10 (SUDS) before you start and check again occasionally whilst you tap. This ensures that you have really cleared the emotional or physical pain. If you are working on a phrase that seems just a bit too far for you right now, then add the phrase "I can imagine that I could…." Or "I am almost there but not quite yet".

There is no pressure to take on the words and phrases in this book; only to use them as a guide. Persistence and being specific will give you good results.

Happy Tapping!
Diane

Abandonment

There may have been times in your life when you have felt abandoned, or have yourself abandoned a person or a situation. These phrases may help you tune in and forgive yourself and others.

Finding the core issues	Finding the words to re-frame
I was abandoned/I abandoned……	I /they did what was right at the time
I was left alone/I left…. behind	
It's very painful to remember	That was then, and this is now
It has affected my whole life	I choose to forgive (him/her/them/me)
I can't ever forgive or forget	
It keeps on happening	There is no reason to let this affect my life
This has left a void in my heart	
I am scarred with this pain	I choose to let this go
I feel scared of this happening again	It will not happen again
	My heart is full of love
	I let the pain go
	I feel safe and loved

Write anything else you think of here:	I love, accept and forgive myself

Abundance

Abundance issues are usually centred around the lack of something; maybe money! You may have to dig a little to find out where these beliefs might have originated, some maybe from childhood.

Finding the core issues	Finding the words to re-frame
I am always poor	I have enough
There is never enough money	There is no lack of anything
I can't have what others have	There is always plenty
I never had anything new as a child	I am abundant with everything I need
Lack of money makes me scared	I am abundant with love
I feel uptight around money	Money flows to me, I am a money magnet!
I hate opening the post	
I don't open bank statements	I am grateful for this abundance
I'm scared that there will never be enough	I love receiving money and good news
	Money is energy and it flows as it's meant to
	The more I give the more I get

Write anything else you think of here:	I love, accept and forgive myself

Addictions

Addictions cover many aspects of life; alcohol, cigarettes, drugs, shopping, gambling, even over eating certain foods like chocolate! Please just concentrate on your issue where I have put dots. …..

Finding the core issues	Finding the words to re-frame
I can't live without….	I know I have to stop this
I have to have…..	My addiction is making me ill
It won't do me any harm	My addiction is costing too much money
My Grandparents….all their life and they were OK	
	It's unfair to my family
It's not hurting anyone else	I am stronger than… .. (it)
I deserve my treat	I want to be free of…… (it)
I work hard, and this is my reward	I know I am better than this and I choose change
I look forward to my…………	
It blocks out the pain/issues in my life	I am beating this ……..now
	I choose to be free of my addiction

Write anything else you think of here:	I love, accept and forgive myself

Allergies

Allergies can be serious so make sure you do this work after understanding the depth of the allergy. If on the other hand you are worried about an intolerance, maybe to food or chemicals, then the words and phrases here may help. Get an allergy test so you know which substances are causing the symptoms.

Finding the core issues	Finding the words to re-frame
I am sneezing all the time	I choose to live without this 'allergy'
My nose runs like a tap	
My eyes are sore and weepy	My body heals itself
I hate this allergy	I send love and healing to every part of my body
This makes me feel ill and tired	
My skin has a rash, I itch….	I listen to my body
I am fed up with this, I hurt	I take care to eat what is right for me
I hate having to be so careful with foods/chemicals	My body understands what I have to do
I feel my life is restricted by this allergy	I choose not to pollute my body with chemicals
Why did this happen to me/poor me	Life if full and has no restrictions
	I accept that my life can change for the better

Write anything else you think of here:	I love, accept and forgive myself

Anger

This is a very powerful emotion and can affect every moment of your life. You may be feeling angry with life in general or something more specific. This can also be an underlying emotion in relationship and career issues.

Finding the core issues	Finding the words to re-frame
This anger feels like………	Anger is a waste of energy
He/she said….and that makes me very angry	Anger will change nothing
	I choose to release my anger
My life is not meant to be like this	I am free of anger and frustration
Nothing goes right for me	I am loved by everyone, I am safe
My partner makes me so cross	I forgive myself for holding this anger
My job is a washout and I hate it	
No matter what I do, it's wrong	I choose to believe I can change
I am ill/in pain and I don't deserve this	My body deserves love and compassion
I have never been loved - I have no real friends	I choose to be free of anger

Write anything else you think of here:	I love, accept and forgive myself

Anxiety

This emotion is one of the most common and often accompanies constant worrying. Some people even invent things to worry about as they are uncomfortable without the familiar feeling of anxiety. It is also part of a 'fear or phobia' emotion, so see that listing as well.

Finding the core issues	Finding the words to re-frame
This anxiety	I see no reason to worry or be anxious
I am worried about everything	
What will happen to me/my family if ? happens	I am taken care of
	Worry is a waste of energy
I can't…..because I am so anxious	I choose to be free of worry and anxiety
I will never be able to cope	
I am unable to do what others do	Being anxious will change nothing
My anxiety stops me from enjoying my life	I can be free of worry
	I choose to think and plan instead of worry
I am deeply unhappy because I worry so	
	I am free of anxiety and at peace
I am unable to think for worry and anxiety	I love my freedom to live and be

Write anything else you think of here:	I love, accept and forgive myself

Bereavement

The loss of a person dear to you is not easy to bear but there are also other bereavements, which create similar pain. These can be the loss of a limb, a breast, a womb, an organ or a pet; all devastating and life changing at the time.

Finding the core issues	Finding the words to re-frame
My pain is indescribable	This loss was inevitable
I hurt, every bit of me, in this despair	Everybody/ thing will pass
	My pain will ease
I will never get over this loss	My loss will become bearable
Life will never be the same again	My loss is not that significant in the great scheme of things
I am finding this really hard	
I can't cope	I choose to accept this
This is not acceptable	I choose to move on with my life
How can I think of anything else?	My life will heal
I will never get over this	I choose to find peace
No one understands how I feel	Life will move on as I get stronger

Write anything else you think of here:	I love, accept and forgive myself

Business and Career Issues

Also see Abundance - Our work takes up a huge part of our lives and can take up an inordinate amount of energy. To be in the right job or career or to have a thriving business will give us contentment, but the reverse gives us pain, anger and anxiety. It is also common to feel lost and unable to focus when things go wrong.

Finding the core issues	Finding the words to re-frame
I am so unhappy at work	I love my job, I do my very best
I am not recognised for my work	It's not important to be recognised
I am unhappy with colleagues	I choose to show love to my colleagues
My business is not doing as well as I hoped	
	I have respect for everyone
No one shows me respect	My business is doing OK
I have no idea why I am doing this	I am passionate about what I do
My whole life is a waste of time	I am truly blessed in this life
I work so hard that I miss out on life	I make time for my family and/recreation
I may go bankrupt – I have such fear	I am abundant with customers
	I attract wealth through my work, with no fear
I am so scared of doing this	

Write anything else you think of here:	I love, accept and forgive myself

Cancer and other serious illnesses

It's not easy to accept illness as part of our path in life. When a medical professional has informed us that we have………….. we believe it. This news will take your energy and positive thoughts away, so use the tapping to re-establish who you really are and think yourself well. Be persistent and tap regularly…three to four times a day may be required.

Finding the core issues	Finding the words to re-frame
Why me? It's not fair	Life is all about learning
It runs in the family, so I expected it	Maybe this is meant for my growth
This is not how my life should be	
I can't stand the pain/discomfort any more	I choose not to accept this like my family did
How do I cope with/tell my family/friends?	I choose to release my pain
	My family and friends support me
What if I die? I'm scared	
It feels like hospital has a revolving door for me	I will only die when I am ready
	I create my own life
I enjoy the attention I get	My …… and my body is healing
People care for me when I'm ill	I am loved and safe
	I find peace in every day

Write anything else you think of here:	I love, accept and forgive myself

Children's behavioral issues

Raising children is not easy and in some cases children have physiological reasons for what is considered 'bad' behaviour. This will often need specialist help but for the majority, children can be helped with EFT; it can be useful to have a soft toy with the points sewn on with buttons for the child to tap on. It is important that parents/carers understand that this is a regular practise until there is noticeable change. For a small child, tap with them and say together the phrases and see if the child will come up with more, for older children they can just be guided until they 'feel' the benefits.

Finding the core issues	Finding the words to re-frame
People say I am naughty	I want to be a good boy/girl
I get lots of attention when I act like this	I know that I am loved
I don't understand what **they** want	I choose to think about what people say to me
I like the angry feelings I get	I know that being angry is not good
I like breaking toys/hitting out	I choose to be fair to others
When I scream it feels good	I can tap to feel good
I am scared of what I do sometimes	I just want to be OK
I feel very lonely	I have many friends
I hate everyone	I love my MUM/DAD/CARER/SIBLINGS

Write anything else you think of here:	I love, accept and forgive myself

Chronic Fatigue Syndrome

This syndrome has the effect of long term tiredness which gets no better with sleep. Many people find it hard to concentrate and therefore are unable to work. The tapping will, in most cases, help alleviate symptoms and gradually assist in an increase of wellness. An alkaline diet may also help.

Finding the core issues	Finding the words to re-frame
I am so tired and exhausted	I accept this tiredness/illness
I find it hard to get out of bed some days	It's part of who I am
Why did this have to happen to me?	Maybe there's a reason-I need to think about that
I ache/hurt all over	I choose to tap away my pains
I feel overwhelmed	I accept this is here now and will go soon
I can't even talk properly/find the right words	I look forward to being better
I need quiet and peace around me	I am grateful for the people who have shown up for me and take care of me
I need to be taken care of	
It's not fair on my family/friends	I am so lucky to be loved

Write anything else you think of here:	I love, accept and forgive myself

Depression

Depression takes many forms, so this list is hardly exhaustive. I have used here the words and phrases that I have come across but please add your own. Do not change medication without your doctor's permission.

Finding the core issues	Finding the words to re-frame
My depression makes me sick	I appreciate and love my body
I feel so low most of the time	I have a chance to choose a better way
No one loves/cares about me anyway	
	I can look to the future again
I have to take medication/drugs just to cope	I have no need of drugs
	I have a positive outlook on life
I have never fitted in	I eat well to feed my brain
I have anger/fear inside me	There is so much I want to do
My life is a waste of time	I start each day with happiness
It's not easy to even get out of bed	I love my family/friends so much
I am letting everyone down	I find peace in my life

Write anything else you think of here:	I love, accept and forgive myself

Fears & Phobias

See also Anxiety. These emotions are similar and once again I can only make some suggestions for the tapping routine. If you have a very severe phobia it may be a good idea to have another person with you, it will help if you feel overwhelmed and help you to check your progress.

Finding the core issues	Finding the words to re-frame
I can't look at/do that	It's only a thought and I am in charge of my thoughts
I refuse to think about it	
I can't bear it. Make it go away	I can picture my fear/phobia with calmness
I shake with fear, I am overwhelmed	
	I value the thought that I am free of this
I've always been like this	
I have to live with it	My fear is leaving me
I am like my Mum (or whoever)	I am calm and peaceful
It may be irrational, but I am scared anyway	I love my life
	I choose to rise above my fear/phobia
I don't ever want to face it	
It's normal not to like…..	There is no need to be scared, I am safe
	I am free to live my life

Write anything else you think of here:	I love, accept and forgive my self

Fibromyalgia

This is a debilitating illness and it sometimes takes doctors time to recognise the symptoms and give appropriate support. There would be a time when you did not have this illness, so go back to that time and replay your life to find the 'trigger' or underlying cause(s).

Finding the core issues	Finding the words to re-frame
Doc says my pains are fibromyalgia, need tablets	I don't have to believe the doctor
I ache all over and I am tired	Maybe I don't need to take drugs for long
I find it hard to do anything	My body can and will heal
My joints hurt	I choose to feel well
I get headaches	I choose not to have pain
I need to sleep, and I can't	I sleep well and feel rested
I am never able to rest	My life is wonderful
This is not the way I wanted my life to be	I choose to be grateful
I can't live like this any more	I live a pain-free life of love

Write anything else you think of here:	I love, accept and forgive myself

Hypertension (high blood pressure)

This set of phrases can be used for low blood pressure and heart conditions as well. It's all about acceptance that your heart, as a pump, will function well for you.

Finding the core issues	Finding the words to re-frame
My blood is under pressure	My blood is pure and runs freely
I am under pressure	I have no pressure to do anything
I am stressed and over worked	There is no stress in my body
My heart is feeling the pressure	I choose to be calm and at peace
I may have to take tablets forever	I help my heart heal
I never expected this	My heart and blood are working for me
I always expected this, it's in the family	I love my life
This is not the way my life should be	I am grateful for my body
I am getting old and ill	I choose to live in health and happiness

Write anything else you think of here:	I love, accept and forgive myself

Insomnia

This can be caused by many external factors like too much light or noise, but the most common is emotional stress which is out of control, fear of the unknown and constant brain activity. Just imagining the tapping when in bed can be a great help.

Finding the core issues	Finding the words. to re-frame
I have so much to think about	I choose peace and calmness
I worry over everything	I release my worries
I can't sleep	I allow my body to relax
I need to rest, I am exhausted	I am rested by the morning
My brain won't stop	I choose to free my mind
I am fearful of......	I have nothing to fear
I am unhappy	I am content with my life
I have so much stress	I release the stress of the day
No one understands me	I am grateful for what I have
	I breathe away my worries and rest

Write anything else you think of here:	I love, accept and forgive myself

Pain Management

Your pain may be ongoing or short lived, but whichever it is, persistence pays! Be specific; "The pain in my big toe on my left foot" for instance. Focus on the pain and give it a rating before you start.

Finding the core issues	Finding the words to re-frame
This pain	I acknowledge this pain
The pain in my……….	My body is telling me something
It's been there……. / forever	I choose to release this pain
It's /it was not my fault	I cast no blame
I never asked for this	I forgive myself anyway
Why me?	There is a reason for this pain
Someone………. caused this pain	I allow my body to heal
I am angry about this pain	I release my anger
This is frustrating	I truly accept my body will heal

Write anything else you think of here:	I love, accept and forgive myself

Relationship Issues

Relationship issues are not just about your partner; they cover parents, family, friends and work colleagues. Be specific when you can and find the words that suit your issues.

Finding the core issues	Finding the words to re-frame
I hate……	I want to forgive
He/She makes me sick	I need forgiveness
I am angry with…. because….	I release my anger and hatred
I can't bear him/her to be near me……	I choose to think differently about…..
He/She must hate me because…..	I realise it was no one's fault
We will just never get on	I know we can start to talk about this
He/She has never liked me	
There is no way I want to talk to….. again	I choose not to hate anyone
	I wish to mend this relationship
I feel so sad that this has happened	I choose to forgive and move on
My life is a mess	I release this pain

Write anything else you think of here:	I love, accept and forgive myself

Stress

This seems to be around in epidemic proportions, whether it is work, relationships, family life or just everyday living. Try taking several deep breaths before and during your tapping session. On the out breath visualise yellow (solar plexus) stress leaving your body.

Finding the core issues	Finding the words to re-frame
Life is so stressful	Life is fun
My life is frantic, and I worry	I choose to slow down my thinking
Why is my life like this? It's not what I want	I create my own reality
I can't seem to make any headway	I can focus on the good things in my life
I feel overwhelmed and out of control	I release my need to control everything
I hate this …….job/person/situation	I allow love back into my life
Things happen that make me panic	I am calm and peaceful
There is too much going on	I take my tasks one at a time
This stress is making me ill	I love my stress-free life

Write anything else you think of here:	I love, accept and forgive myself

Trauma (PTSD) Post Traumatic Stress Disorder

Your trauma could be anything from a minor car accident that left you too scared to drive, to a very serious incident or life-threatening situation. It could be something that seems major to you, but is not thought of as very serious by others.

Finding the core issues	Finding the words to re-frame
I can't bear to think about it	I don't have to think about it
I don't want to remember the details	I choose to let it go
I see it in my dreams/thoughts	I free my body of this emotional pain
It keeps on coming back to me	I accept it was not my fault
I was/am in profound shock	I forgive …..(others)
It was all so dreadful	That was then, and this is now
No one will ever understand	I let this baggage go
Talking about it gives me……	I am loved and cared for
I want it to stop	I allow this trauma to leave me
	I choose to feel peace

Write anything else you think of here:	I love, accept and forgive myself

Weight and Food Issues

If you have issues around food or your weight, you may be obsessed by meal times, what to eat and then feel guilty for eating too much. Like everything this has underlying issues, you may need to dig deep to uncover them. My tip is to start with childhood memories and see what that brings up.

For the overweight

Finding the core issues	Finding the words to re-frame
I am fat, and I hate my body	I desire to be slimmer for the good of my health
I love to eat, then I am consumed with guilt	I choose to release all guilt
I am OK with my fat sometimes	I choose to be in control of my thoughts
My family are overweight, so it's in my genes	I release this obsession with food
This way of life may kill me	I feed my body when and what it needs
I can't stop eating, I have no control	I listen to my body and feel the fullness
No one loves this fat person that I am	Each day is a positive day
I start each day with good intentions and then blow it	I'm happy to be the slim person I choose to be
This is affecting all areas of my life	I am doing the very best I can

Write anything else you think of here:	I love, accept and forgive myself

For those suffering from bulimia or anorexia

Tapping will reinforce your self-esteem and self-love.

Finding the core issues	Finding the words to re-frame
I need/have to be thin	Being this thin is not good for my health
I love to eat but I can't	
The thought of food is repulsive	I need to eat to live
Food makes me fat and fat is not OK	Food is my body's fuel
I am only loved when I am thin	I only eat enough for a healthy body
I am in control of me and my food	
Control is a big issue for me	I am still in control when I eat more
I hate my body – I feel overwhelming guilt	I respect my body and listen to its needs
I can't stop this obsession	
How can food have such a hold over my thoughts and emotions?	I choose to change my life and release guilt
	I love my body, whatever shape it is
	I am loved for me not my body

Write anything else you think of here:	I love, accept and forgive myself

God grant me the serenity to accept the people I cannot change, the courage to change the one I can, and the wisdom to know it's me.
Author unknown, variation of an excerpt from "The Serenity Prayer" by Reinhold Neibuhr

The copyright to this book is owned by Diane Holliday who is the creator and author

Diane is an Advanced EFT Practitioner, registered with AAMET

More details about Diane and contact information can be found on her web site www.dianeholliday.co.uk

Printed in Great Britain
by Amazon